Martin BAUER

Maternity

Preparation guide to childbirth

To be put in the hands of future moms, future dads, families and helpers!

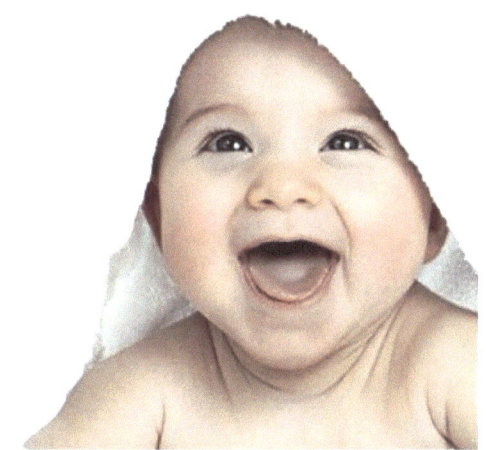

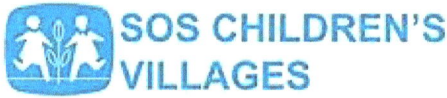

Half of the benefits from this book will be donated to SOS Children's Villages, a non-governmental organization that provides children and families around the world with a home and a caring education. For more information, visit:

https://www.sos-childrensvillages.org/

To my Dad, who is watching us from above and looks after Gabrielle.

Special Thanks

I wish to thank from the deepest of my heart all those who accompanied me in maternity and parenting and made possible the writing of this work.

To my dear husband, my companion, my sidekick, my friend, my half in this wonderful adventure of parenthood.

To my big family, all the women and all the children who are part of it and made me gain experience before finally becoming a mother in my turn.

To all the parents I had the chance to meet throughout my journey and who brought me advice and kindness.

To you, reader, who has taken on yourself to trust me, I hope that this book will bring you support and information.

To you all, this book is yours, I hope it will accompany you the best way possible in this fabulous adventure which is parenting.

Foreword

While I was having a difficult pregnancy that forced me to keep in bed, I fed myself - as much as my cognitive abilities diminished by the hormonal storm allowed me – with books about pregnancy, preparation for childbirth, and parenting. I was terrified of experiencing this dangerous experience of giving birth, with the lot of questions it could imply.

I remember that keeping myself informed and trying to prepare for any eventuality helped me particularly to overcome my concerns and agree to best get ready for this inevitable experience.

This book is a support for compulsory courses in France in preparation for entering the maternity ward. It is a collection of advice and good practices offered by midwives, obstetricians, childcare assistants and experienced parents. It is not proposed to you in place of the compulsory courses, but will allow you to prepare them, to raise certain questions which you will then be able to note on the pages proposed for this purpose, to ask them then to the midwives. Or simply take notes during class. It is both very useful during preparation to birth and can also serve as information medium for the future dad or any accompanying person. It is a tool for work and reflection on your delivery. Make it yours, underline, fluoride, comment in the margins! This book is in its first edition, so do not hesitate to propose me improvements on my Twitter account.

Finally, half of the benefits of this book will be donated to a non-governmental organization serving children, which I also propose to elect on my Twitter account. [* Author's Note: the NGO selected is SOS Children's Villages, more information on https://www.sos-childrensvillages.org/]

Do not hesitate to recommend this book around you! I wish you an excellent preparation for the most beautiful adventure in the history of humanity. It's your trip. Ready for takeoff!

Summary

Table of Contents

Course 1: Preliminary Information

Anatomy of pregnancy

During a normal pregnancy, the baby moves freely in the womb until the 5th or 6th month, when the uterus reaches its maximum size. The fetus (embryo until the 3rd month) can then be in the head down position for the future exit.

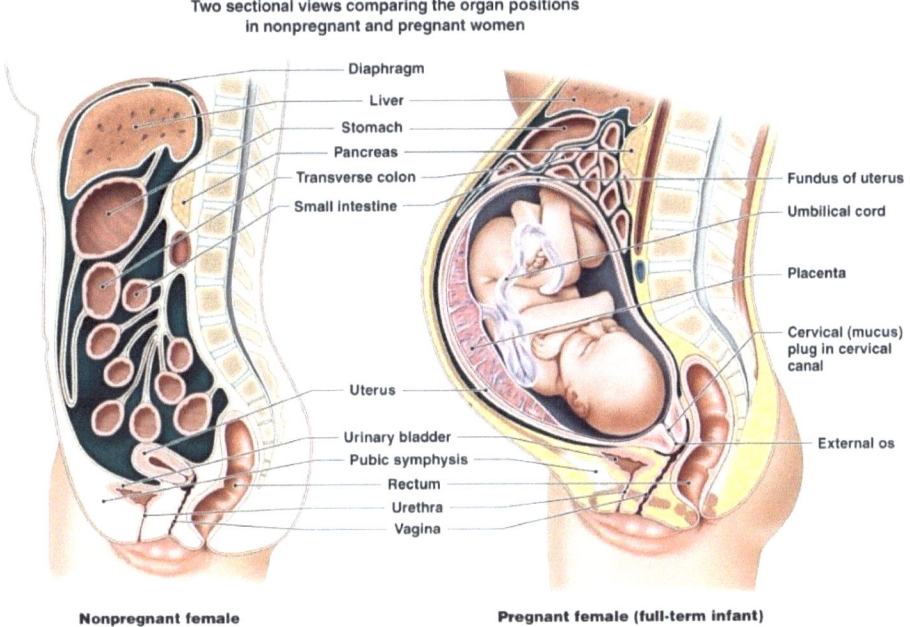

Two sectional views comparing the organ positions in nonpregnant and pregnant women

Diaphragm
Liver
Stomach
Pancreas
Transverse colon
Small intestine
Fundus of uterus
Umbilical cord
Placenta
Cervical (mucus) plug in cervical canal
Uterus
Urinary bladder
Pubic symphysis
Rectum
Urethra
Vagina
External os

Nonpregnant female

Pregnant female (full-term infant)

© 2011 Pearson Education, Inc.

The position is final in the 9th month, when the future infant has all the trouble to move in the womb. In the case of a sitting position, it is preferable that the mother tries to reposition the baby with the help of an osteopath, for example.

Anatomy of childbirth

During labor, the contractions cause the dilatation and then the collapse of the cervix, to facilitate the passage of the baby for its release in the open air.

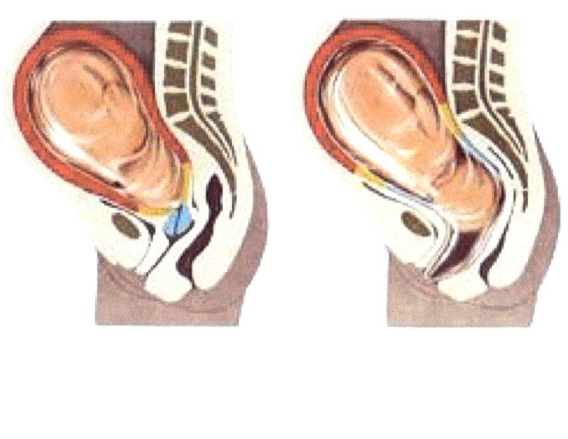

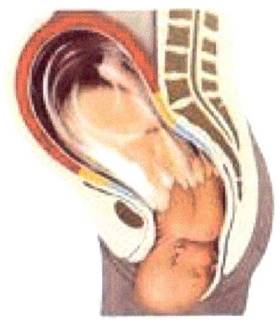 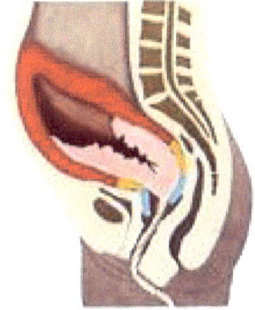

As the neck collapses, the water pocket eventually breaks through for the infant to exit. When the baby is out, the last contractions cause the expulsion of the placenta. It is called afterbirth or delivering.

Birth Project

The birth plan is developed during pregnancy by the mother or both parents. It includes the desire or not to appeal to the epidural, the place of birth, hospital, clinic or birthing center (or home), delivery method, classic, balloon, chair, pool ... we also choose the position, etc. Inform the nursing staff about your project and it will do everything to satisfy it. You can also talk to them in advance to check its feasibility. Finally, the maternity hospitals offer guides and various documentation that can serve as support for the implementation of your project, some even have "pink boxes" or "maternity boxes" including various offers: do not hesitate to ask for them as soon as possible. This birth plan is your connection with the maternity ward. For more information, please go to "Building Your Birth Project" on page 47.

Notes

Course 2: Start of labor and associated postures

When the time comes to give birth to the baby, the contractions inform the mother that the delivery is near. The mother may have painless contractions throughout her pregnancy that manifest as hardening of the belly due to the contracting uterus. Labor contractions are more important and painful. The arrival of childbirth can also be expressed by a loss of water (the amniotic fluid pocket is pierced) but is more rare.

Case 1: Work Contractions - Frequent (in 2 out of 3 women)

Not to mention "false alarm", contractions must be painful, each one is of the same intensity and occur every 5 minutes for 1 hour and a half to 2 hours minimum.

➔ Then we go to the maternity hospital after these 2 hours

How to avoid "false alarms"?

Start with a 20-minutes nap or a warm bath (be careful, do not be alone at home if you lose consciousness due to heat)

→ If the contractions subside or lose their regularity, this is a false alarm

How to "use" contractions?

Walking in or around the place where you are with long inspirations, to refocus the baby in relation to the pelvis to ensure optimal passage and avoid additional pain and risk due to improper centering.

Work postures

In the case of contractions, it is strongly recommended to increase the effectiveness of the centering by regular exercises to 2 with the dad.

For example, the mother can press both hands against a wall to stretch her back, while the dad helps her stretch her back or the mass of the tailbone toward her shoulders.

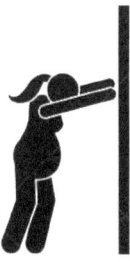

The woman can also hang herself from a doorknob (or the man) and sit in a vacuum to stretch her back and free her

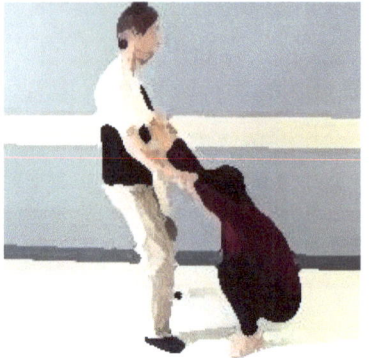

back   and   pelvis.

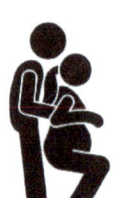

She can also press her upper body on a 4-legged Pilates ball while the man is massaging her back, or stretching her shoulders and neck in the direction of the coccyx to the back of the neck.

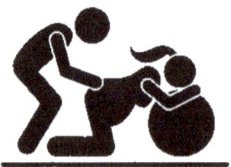

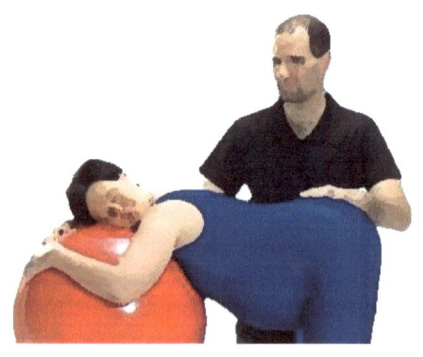

Case 2: Rupture of the water pocket - rare (in 1 in 3 women)

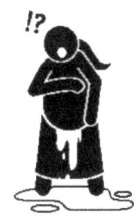 As soon as the water pocket is broken, we have 1h to 1h30 to go to the clinic. Take the time to take a shower (be careful not to bath, because the baby is now in an open system and therefore runs a risk of contamination or infection which is dangerous for him). Take the time to change clothes, and beware, the amniotic fluid continues to renew itself, and to flow down: do not forget to wear for example sanitary towels for your comfort.

Notes

Course 3: Respiration and relaxation

In case of contractions, deep breathing (inhale for 5 seconds while inflating the floating ribs and then relying on the perineum, and then exhale for 10 seconds and gradually close the perineum and abdominals) allows optimal centering of the baby with the pelvis opening.

Simple and effective exercise of centering the baby by breathing for the exit:
1. Kneel down and rest your buttocks on your heels. Your hands are placed flat on the floor in front of you so as to adopt an unobstructed and comfortable position. Keep your back straight, your torso open and your shoulders low.

2. Breathe deeply by opening the coccyx and floating ribs for 5 seconds. You must feel this opening in the back and on the flanks.

3. Hold a second.

4. Visualize your perineum like a diamond whose vertices are attached to your tailbone, your pubic area and on both sides of your vagina.

5. When exhaling, visualize that the vertices of this diamond are getting closer in one point. Exhale for 10 seconds until your abdominals are down.

6. Inhale again by opening the tops of the rhombus and opening coccyx and floating ribs. Reproduce the exercise 5 times in a row.

In case of panic, deep breathing coupled with a simple exercise of mindfulness can evacuate stress, find a little serenity and focus.

Simple exercise of mindfulness:

1. Sit comfortably cross-legged or in a chair with your feet flat on the floor, put your hands on your thighs, close your eyes if you wish.

2. Breathe calmly while attempting deep breathing without forcing.

3. Take the time to observe the path of air in your body, feel the way inspiration and exhalation move it slightly. Inhale and exhale slowly and smoothly while doing the diamond visualization exercise if you do not feel the air going anywhere.

4. Now imagine a soft, warm light at the top of your head. This light will gradually descend over breaths throughout your body. Feel your head invaded, then down the back of your neck, then spread over your shoulders and cross your collarbones. It is now entering your back muscles. The whole of your upper body is now bathed in this soft, soothing and warm light. Take the time to feel its softness and warmth in every part of your body that it enters and do not go to the next part of the body until you feel the heat.

5. Take advantage of the passage of light in your body to identify if a limb or area is painful or tense. If so, take the time to welcome this pain, to observe it, to analyze it, to understand it. Gently pulse the light to soften this area. Breathe deeply and gently into this area so that it relaxes its painful constraints.

6. You will let the light gradually penetrate your back to the lumbar, then impregnate your torso and the entire length of your arms. Your entire rib cage is bathed in the light: your lungs and diaphragm are completely free and your heart beats to the rhythm of your mind bathing from your head in this delicate light.

7. The light now penetrates your last vertebrae, and with them your last ribs: it will finally gently invade the habitat of your baby. Your baby feels this light because it also goes through your cord: it is now connected to your heart and

your mind, you enjoy it to communicate all your love and kindness.

8. Most of your body is now bathed in the light. We are now going to help her to move to a very important part for your body: your whole pelvis, your perineum and your legs. You feel the light pass from the last vertebrae into your coccyx. Below your baby, she enters the highest part of your perineum, the one that holds your anus. It is the one that will hold the rest of your body during childbirth. Then it enters your cervix, which will open slowly under the effect of contractions during delivery. You can then welcome and accompany this movement (especially if you do this exercise during work).

9. Then the light enters the second stratum of your perineum, the one that directs the opening of your vagina, then in the first stratum that holds your urinary orifice: you consider these two strata with a great benevolence, because you will have to relearn them to function properly after delivery.

10. Finally the light pours gently into your hips, then your thighs, your knees, your legs, your ankles and finally to the end of your feet. You allow it to warm gently all these parts of your forelimb, to relieve them to support your whole body and gently soften them.

11. All your body is now bathed in the light. You enjoy for a few breaths this sweet heat and this new well-being. Relax and let your whole body breathe through the light. Then slowly open the eyes.

Notes

Course 4 : During the work

Workflow Attention, a "false alarm" can be calmed by a hot bath or 20 min - 1 nap.

The contractions should be of the same intensity and take place every 5 minutes since 2am. You may be in a pre-work situation if your cervical opening is less than 4 centimeters. The average work lasts from 8 hours to 12 hours, but is usually longer for a first delivery. The delivery itself, which follows the work phase, lasts between 15 minutes and 1 hour, the average duration being around 30 minutes.

Recommandations

Before arriving, drink a sweet and non-acidic drink (e.g. a sweet fruit juice, a syrup), eat lightly. Indeed, it is forbidden in many countries like France to eat or drink during the work in case of need of anesthesia.

Epidural

This analgesia is done on a cervical opening niche of 4 to 8 centimeters. The effects are felt after 15 minutes and last 2 hours renewable by reinjection (and extend the working time of about 2 hours). It helps to soften the pain of labor and delivery without removing sensations, allowing the future mother to make the most out of her contractions.

Be careful, you must know that your baby is also receiving the product of the epidural. In addition, the epidural will often force you to give birth in a supine position, which we will see, is the least indicated for your baby and for your perineum. We recommend that you talk to your midwife about this.

Finally, the epidural is contraindicated in case of fever, blood platelet count too low or tattoo on the area to bite!

Notes

Course 5 : Active labor

The pushing stage is from the beginning of delivery, after the labor phase, when the cervix is at optimal dilation (8 to 10 centimeters) and the "need to push" is felt (like a want to go to the saddle).

Breathing

When the dilation of the cervix is complete, you can start pushing, because the contractions alone will not be enough to expel the baby.

At the time of the contraction, inhale deeply through the nose, and then adopt one of two pushing techniques.

-   **Technique 1 :** At the moment of contraction, exhale gently as if you were blowing into a balloon while pushing; (may not be presented in class)

-   **Technique 2 :** Block your breathing and push while the lungs are still filled with air. (This allows less space for the baby and facilitates his exit - presented in class)

The first technique is more serene and limits the tears, while the second pushes more on the perineum and will generate a longer rehabilitation. However, if one of them does not work for you, test the other. Every woman is

29

different and will find the push technique that suits her best. The important thing is to train as much as possible in the techniques and the thrust positions in order to naturally find the automatisms at the time of delivery.

In order not to exhaust yourself, think about resting and catching your breath between each contraction.

During the course, it was presented to make several pushes by contraction: 1st deep breath for 5 seconds by the nose, blocking 10 seconds, actuation of the abdominals, rise, fast expiration, then immediate inspiration by the mouth, to renew 3 times.

Posture

The posture to be taken to give birth depends on your preferences and your birth plan. For this, it is important to test several positions in advance and to train on those that are best for you, in order to obtain there again, the automatisms necessary for the good progress of the delivery. If you and your partner have decided to share this birthing event, you can train for two, it will greatly simplify the work of the mother.

Here are the most famous postures below.

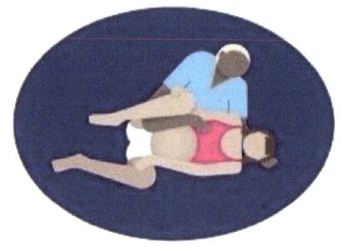

Lying on the side: posture traditionally used in Great Britain but little known in France. It is very useful to free the pelvis and facilitate the passage of the baby while allowing the mother to rest.

Squatting : compatible with giving birth in the pool, the squatting position is considered the most natural to allow the baby to go out. A variant can make you

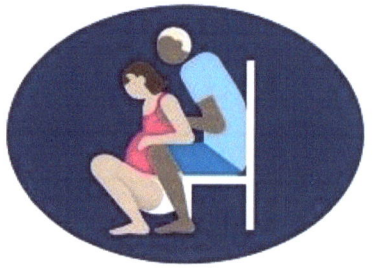

give birth in a delivery chair that will simplify the work of midwives and allow you to rest at times.

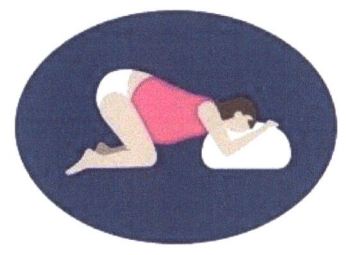 **On all fours:** also compatible with the project of delivery in swimming pool, the four-legged position can free your pelvis, according to your morphology, and avoid many constraints on the perineum. It facilitates the work of the midwives who then take their place behind you.

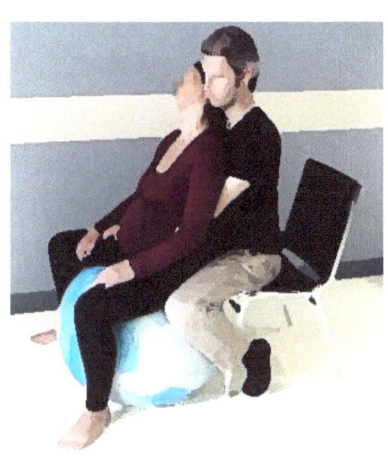 Some postures of collaborative work with the future dad can also be used for childbirth. Do not hesitate to talk to your midwife. Working in pairs makes the delivery experience stronger for both parents while avoiding the maximum of pain for the mother-to-be. Prospective parents must train to the maximum before the crucial date to win together automatisms because the reflection will be put to severe test by the

pains at this precise moment. The training will also reassure both parents. Depending on the birth plan chosen, it is recommended that both parents work on their forelegs (legs) in relaxation and endurance, especially for the father.

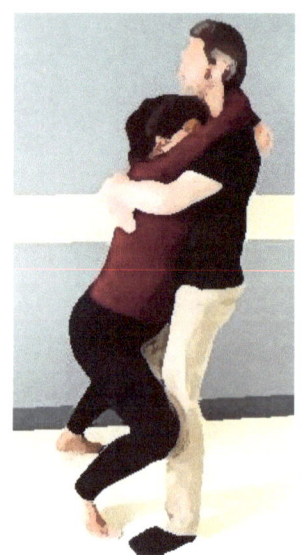

Here, a work posture where the future father massages the future mother by checking the position of her back. This posture can be resumed on all fours during delivery,

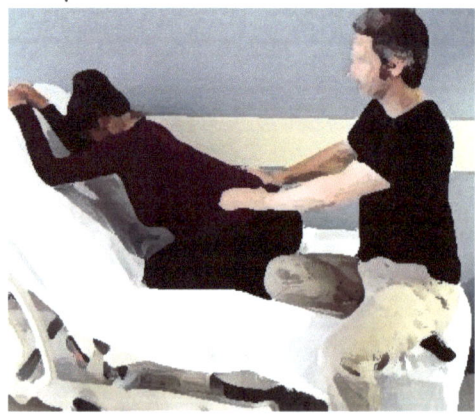

but the father will then shift to the side to leave the place behind the young mother to midwives. (And avoid having in view the passage of the baby which could schok him). The posture indicated in class is often an elongated posture as in the following picture where the man stands behind the woman and pulls his knees towards him during the push, (here, the man is not behind the woman, he can still get on the delivery table behind the woman and place a cushion between them).

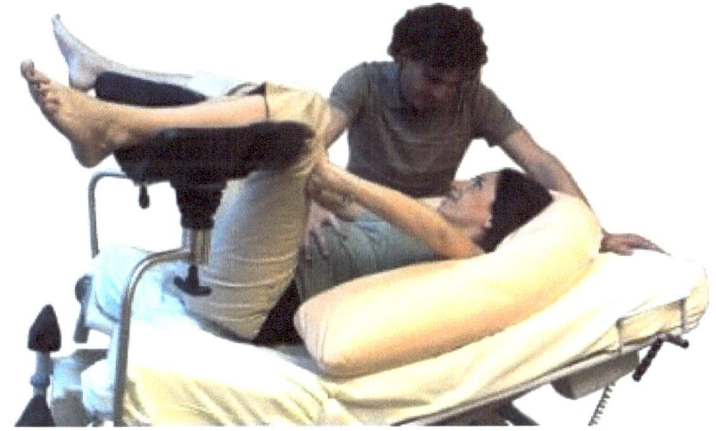

This historical posture simplifies the work of midwives but is completely inappropriate for your perineum or the passage of your baby. It also causes a lot more tears, but will probably be adopted in a hospital or clinic that does not practice natural childbirth if you do not have a birth plan or if you have not trained at other positions.

Notes

Course 6 : Breastfeeding

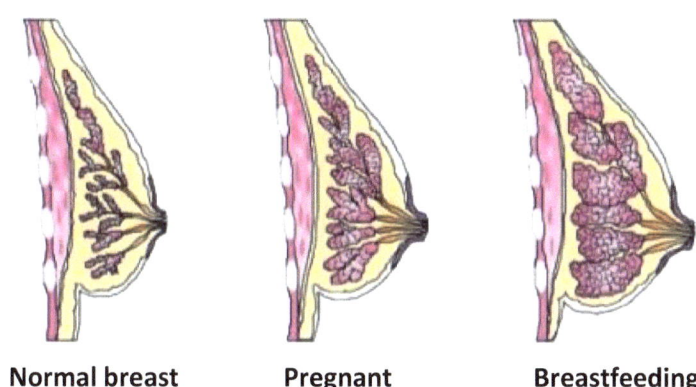

| **Normal breast** | **Pregnant** | **Breastfeeding** |

Lactating cells are the milk-throat cleansers. The lactation hormones are prolactins (for production) and oxytocin (for ejection). The infant will have for reflexes the burrowing (to look for the breast) then the suction (to draw and to suck the milk). It is the suction that causes milk to be produced in the breast.

From 1 to 3 days, the milk is colostrum (first milk, translucent yellow or orange) filled with antibodies and very important to transmit to the baby even if breastfeeding is not envisaged. From about 3 days (this may be more), the definitive milk appears. It is necessary to ensure that the baby, during his first weeks, makes 8 to 15 feedings a day of minimum 10 minutes of suction and active swallowing.

→ So make sure that he sucks as often as possible to feed and to activate the mother's milk production (it is also a training for the baby, the mother and the dad). If you do not plan to breastfeed, it is recommended to ensure a "welcome breastfeeding" so that your baby can benefit from colostrum, which will cleanse the digestive system of the remains of his intrauterine life and improve his immunity. If, on the other hand, your project is to breastfeed, it is recommended to promote the portage and in particular the skin-to-skin which will favor your lactation and the reflexes of search of your baby. This will also aim to reduce the baby's crying and reassure him.

The baby usually loses up to 10% of its weight on the first day (loss of meconium, edema, etc.). It is important that the weight regain is done before the 4th day, for a weight gain of about 150 grams per week.

At the beginning of your baby's life, you will be advised to avoid "pleasure" feedings (that is to say without swallowing or nutrition), as this tires the newborn without allowing him to feed himself and resume forces → then stimulate sucking by tickling the baby on the cheeks or under the chin for 10 to 15 minutes of proper drinking.

Postures

In order to ensure an efficient and painless suckling, the baby's gums must press on the edges of the areola of the breast, as shown in the following diagram.

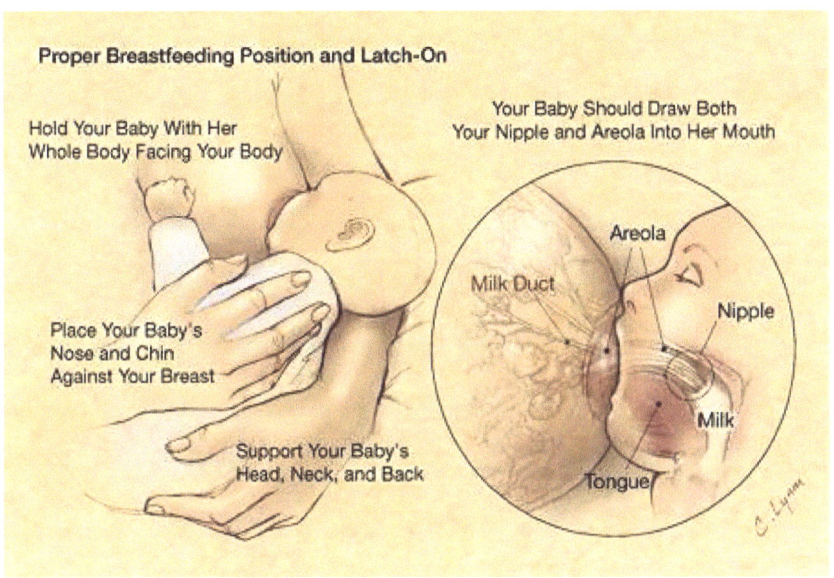

The most popular postures for breastfeeding are as follows:

Each posture has its advantages and each breastfeeding mom will have his or her favorite postures. For example, the elongated or rugby balloon postures will allow you to rest during a long breastfeeding. The Opposite-craddle will be useful at the beginning of breastfeeding, while the baby will need both to be trained to adopt an adequate position and during all the period during which he will not be able to maintain his head all alone. The Craddle, the most classic, will ensure you can interact with your baby with your free hand (caresses, games, etc.). Breastfeeding represents serious benefits for the health of the mother (natural regulation of the weight, reduction of the risk of breast cancer, ...) and the baby (better development of the metabolism and psychomotor development).

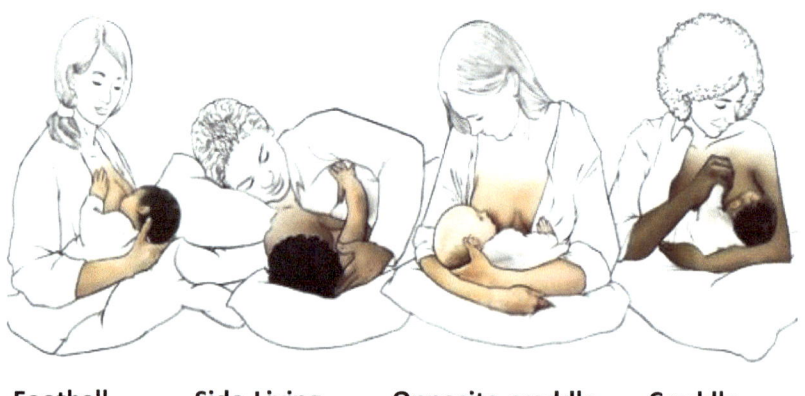

Football   **Side-Liying**   **Opposite-craddle**   **Craddle**

Signs of awakening (when to breastfeed the baby?)

All occasions are good for breastfeeding your baby. At first, he does not know how to express his hunger, especially since he was constantly fed into the womb. Also, it is very important to breastfeed as often as possible and stimulate him as soon as he is awoken.

Baby feeding cues (signs)

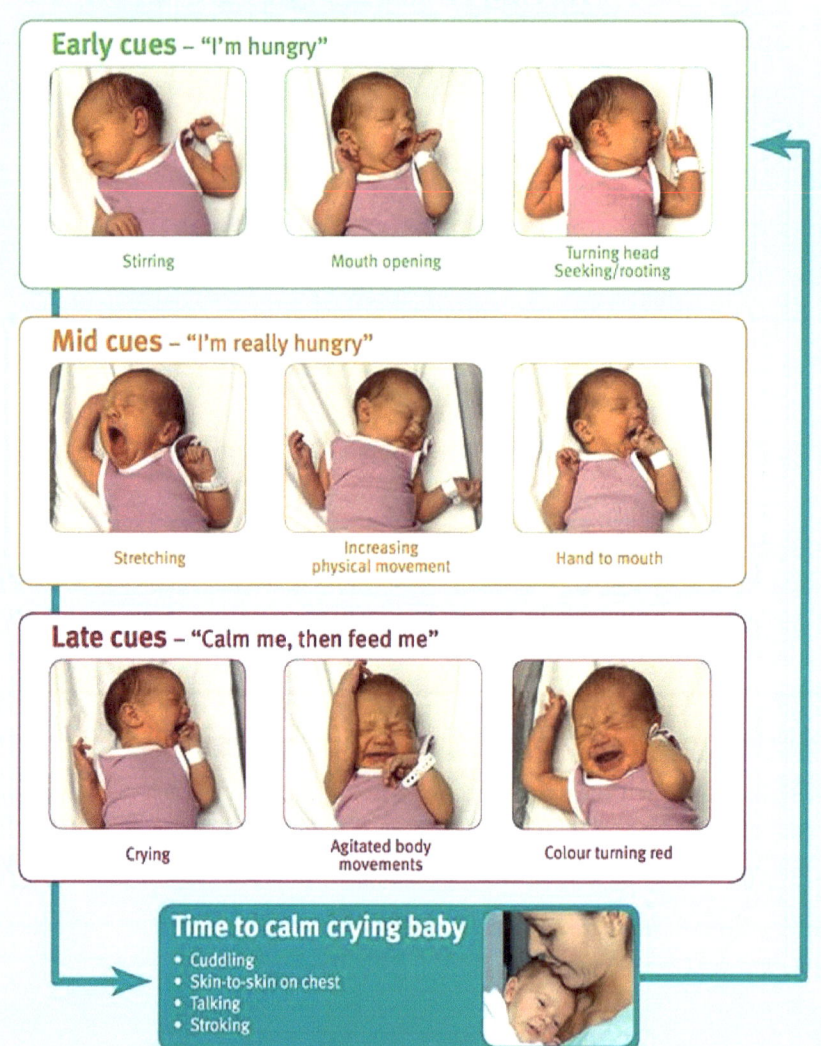

Early cues – "I'm hungry"

Stirring

Mouth opening

Turning head
Seeking/rooting

Mid cues – "I'm really hungry"

Stretching

Increasing
physical movement

Hand to mouth

Late cues – "Calm me, then feed me"

Crying

Agitated body
movements

Colour turning red

Time to calm crying baby
- Cuddling
- Skin-to-skin on chest
- Talking
- Stroking

Notes

Course 7: Medicalization of childbirth

This is the course of explanation of the epidural: although the epidural itself is only the injection of a painkiller, it requires an anesthesia to facilitate the injection of this painkiller, and you will have to give birth while being laid, having an extra catheter in the back (in addition to the one you are carrying on the arm). It is also for this reason, with the cesarean section, that it is forbidden in France and in other countries to eat during the hours of work preceding the delivery, for safety. It is recognized that the epidural removes the pain of childbirth without removing the sensations, while lengthening the duration of the labor. However, each woman will have a different feeling and it is necessary to know the consequences of the choice of the epidural for the mother and the baby, in all kindness and serenity. The future mother who is afraid of the pain but also the consequences for herself and her child will be able to learn about alternative methods of pain prevention, such as hypnosis, for example.

For caesarean section (1 out of 5 births): 2 specific cases

Scheduled caesarean

It is indicated in case of too narrow pelvis or contraindication to vaginal delivery. The delivery is scheduled and the entry in the clinic is the day before. The father can attend the delivery and will be the first to skin-to-skin with the baby while the mother will be in intensive care and then in the recovery room.

Emergency Cesarean

If the baby's heartbeat proves that he can no longer stand the work, the mother is bleeding too much or if the baby is suffocated by the too tight umbilical cord around his neck, it is convenient to the emergency cesarean section, the mother is placed in the operating room and the father is not allowed to attend the operation. It is nevertheless he who will still make the first skin-to-skin.

Exceeding the term date

The respect of the date of term is very important, because 15 days after this date, the calcification of the skull of the infant (process of ossification of the different parts of the skull) will start its process, preventing hence its passage and a vaginal delivery, and present a real risk to his survival and his mother's. In this case, it is a question of preventing the clinic or the chosen place of childbirth and to follow up every 2 days until 10 days, when the oxytocin injection delivery will be triggered. The delivery will then proceed in a normal way.

Notes

Course 8 : Back home

The return back to home is usually done after 4 days of maternity. It is possible to call a midwife during the first month at home, or to be prescribed a daily follow-up, or a lighter one. You may also be prescribed vitamins for the mother and child, as well as all the elements necessary for the care of the cord. Finally, in case of difficult breastfeeding, you can have a breast pump (preferably electric) prescribed to help activate lactation.

Medical monitoring

During the first month, the baby can be followed and weighed weekly by a midwife, then a meeting with the pediatrician (or family doctor) should be scheduled at 1 month, then 2 months to perform the first mandatory vaccines. The child should have a monthly follow up for 1 year, where will be monitored its normal development. The young mother will be able to take advantage of it to ask for advice and recommendations. The mother must schedule an appointment with the obstetrician or her usual gynecologist at 1 month and a half or 2 months after birth, to plan the perineal reeducation that will last on an average of 10 sessions of 1 hour.

Return of menstrual periods

The return of menstrual periods is normally the return of the cycle of the woman: the uterus bleeds during practically the whole month following the delivery (regeneration of the uterus), then the bleeding diminishes and stops after one month and the new menstrual normally appear at the end of the 2nd month postpartum, except for the breastfeeding mother who will not have her periods until about 6 months to 18 months after the delivery, or even the end of breastfeeding. Two months after the childbirth, you can start pelvic reeducation and then slowly and ste-by-step come back to sport by walking, swimming or cycling.

Infant colic

In cases of colic, more frequent in the case the baby is fed with artificial milk (for the breastfed infant, they may never occur or stop as early as the 2nd month), take the baby in skin to skin or massage his belly counter clockwise. To help you, see noon in front of you, your hand will be turning on the baby's belly so that they reach noon on the left and leave noon on the right.

« Making his nights »

When a baby is "making his nights", it means he can sleep for 6 hours without waking up. This is usually done between 3 to 4 months when the baby has doubled its birth weight. If after 4 months the baby is still not sleeping, consult an osteopath, it could be a problem of placement of the bones of the skull.

Travelling

By plane, you must breastfeed the baby on the ascent and descent. Nothing in theory contravenes air travel, although any form of travel is not recommended for the well-being of the baby who is not yet one year old. In case of travel, it is also necessary to make sure that the baby is well hydrated and has a good body temperature.

Notes

Optional course 1: Building your birth project

As about the 7th month of pregnancy, the midwife will talk to you about your "birth plan" and how to prepare it for the nursing staff just before the delivery. However, the creation of this project begins with the positive pregnancy test. It mainly concerns how you want to give birth, but can also have an impact on the progress of your pregnancy. In the detail of the birth plan, you designate the place of delivery, choose the medical methods and evaluate if they are possible in your case, as well as the progress of the maternity.

Place
The choice of several birthing places is offered to you:

- At the hospital (chosen in France in the case of low resources and at-risk births): it is necessary in this case to apply for care at the hospital at the time of the positive test or at the latest at the 3rd month to get a place in.

- In clinic (model chosen most of the time for the flexibility and the diversity of services offered including those of the hospital): the clinics can notably propose natural birthing methods limiting the pain, as well as services close to those of the hotels, which can accommodate the father and the family.

- In birth center (or birthing house, chosen for the natural and reassuring aspect of the care): it is necessary in this case to present no risk to the delivery, including a presentation at the exit of the baby by the head, the presentation by the seat being able to provocate risks for the mother and the child. The concept of these houses is becoming more and more popular in European countries and is increasingly being offered as complementary services to clinics or hospitals, allowing direct access to operating theaters in the event of unforeseen risks.

- At home, a very rare case (1% of cases), requiring a registered midwife and a particular preparation, but which can ensure total peace of mind for parents worried about having to go through the hospital environment, and wishing to maintain control over their birth project.

Method

The method of general delivery will be mainly dictated by your state of health. For example, future mothers or babies with specific health risks (cardiovascular diseases, diabetes, need for operation at birth, etc.) should be given special monitoring during pregnancy and validate with their caregiver a level of care that will have to be ensured. For this purpose we often speak of level 1, level 2 or level 3 or 4 hospitals for the heaviest care. In terms of equipment used (monitors, suction cups, forceps, ...), it is possible that the obstetrician in charge of your delivery (in this case, it may be the obstetrician on duty) must make decisions on the spot according to the evolution of childbirth itself. This is also true for episiotomy, if a complex tear is emerging (1 in 5 cases). If you want to avoid an episiotomy as much as possible, the preparation during pregnancy is even more important: the facilitation of the passage of your baby does not only depend on its size, but especially on your flexibility which can be reinforced by yoga classes, Pilates, Tai chi and Qi gong. The elasticity of your flesh can be ensured by a good hydration. Finally, your control of breathing, delivery position and ejection can greatly simplify the passage of the newborn by minimizing pain. This can also be reinforced by mindfulness meditation exercises. The choice of your birthing method is therefore often on time, but you can influence this method as much as possible by preparing yourself as much as possible, physically, mentally and spiritually.

Stackeholders

In general, the care team will consist of one or more midwives, an obstetrician (for infant discharge and surgical care), an anesthesiologist where appropriate, and one or more caregivers. In order to reassure the mother-to-be and help her give birth to her baby, it is recommended that she surround herself with one or more companions with whom she will have trained beforehand at the delivery positions. Nowadays, fatherhood is more and more established and developed in men, it is often recommended that the father be the first helper, so both parents discover together their parenthood and prepare for it together, which makes the preparation even more effective for everyone. However, if it is impossible for the father to be present at the birth, the young mother can surround herself with family members or trusted ones.

Anesthesia

The epidural consists of the diffusion of an analgesic by intravenous, after local anesthesia. In theory, it has the advantage of limiting the pain without removing the sensation of passage, which would allow the young mother to ensure nevertheless the pushing stage. The disadvantage is that the epidural tends to greatly extend the duration of work ... and therefore painful sensations, discomfort and risks for the baby. In addition, the baby receiving all that is inoculated to his mother, he also receives an elevated dose of product at birth, and will potentially have fewer reflexes, including breastfeeding. Many pregnant women wonder about the need for an epidural. Indeed, for a first child, it is difficult to assess the level of pain in advance, as well as the level of acceptance of this pain. Many women are also afraid in advance of the feeling of this pain, especially when they have heard about it from their elders in this experience. To this, many midwives say that epidurals are only practiced in societies in economically highly developed countries, and that, as a result, the overwhelming majority of women in the world give birth without an epidural. You should know that the least bearable pain is not during delivery but during labor. During delivery, the woman is active and focuses on the effective push. Although the pain is overwhelming, the importance of allowing the baby to go out quickly is more important and occupies much of the mental space of the woman. If the pain related to contractions and dilation of the cervix are still bearable, then the epidural will be useless, even cumbersome (a catheter and its pipe in the back, associated with an automatically lying position, is the least comfortable for the push and the riskier for the infant) and counterproductive. To this end, many women, after having had their first epidural birth, choose to give up for the next ones. Indeed, the effects of the pain can also be inhibited by prior training (flexibilisation of the pelvis and visualization by meditation of the passage of the baby) and choice of an adequate working position and delivery.

Position

As we have seen before, the position is of paramount importance in the smooth running of labor and delivery. The final choice of your preferred positions should be made in the last trimester of pregnancy, when the pregnant woman is at her maximum size, so that she can identify areas of physical constraints, comfort zones and clearances, and that her partner can also accompany her in the best work and childbirth. In general, the laid position often presented in class is the worst for the comfort of the mother and the passage of the infant: in this position, nevertheless more comfortable for the nursing staff, the pelvis collapses, hindering the passage of the baby and the perineum is subject to constraints that can make rehabilitation more sluggish and painful, as well as the most important inconveniences caused (strong urinary or faecal incontinence, organ descents, etc.). It is therefore necessary to identify the best work and delivery positions and to check their compatibility with the work of the nursing staff and the choice of your method and place of delivery. For example, it will be difficult to give birth lying in the pool, however the four-legged position is quite appropriate for this environment. To go further, you can choose your working positions by studying the types of contractions (ventral, renal, etc.) and the attitude and the breathing to adopt, as well as the massages that can be done by the father to simplify the work

Postpartum development

When your baby is finally placed in your arms, you are at the same time caught between the happiness of welcoming this little being and the need to discover it, and the need to ensure its survival, once assured by the placenta during the intrauterine life. You want both to rest your efforts and your emotions while finally enjoying moments of calm with your baby. However, you enter a period of several days at the maternity ward, where the caregiver will come almost every hour to care for you and your baby, check if the baby is well fed (breastfeeding can then get very stressful for the mother whereas it should consist of wonderful moments), weigh the baby, take blood, but also give you baby care classes, offer paid services (in some clinics), and where your relatives can also visit you. Added to this is the fact that you sleep badly (either because your baby, disoriented by this new environment, cries, or because you are not accustomed to sleeping in hospital, or because your body is suffering the effects of possible surgical interventions, or even all this at once), and that the food of the establishment is not at your convenience, but also potentially other disappointments and dysfunctions related to these establishments receiving a lot of public. In the case the young mother remains alone in the maternity with her baby without the father being able to share their evenings or their nights, this loneliness can also weigh on the psychological state of the mother.

This accumulation can then transform what should be the most beautiful experience of a lifetime into a real nightmare for the mother weakened by pregnancy, childbirth and the hormonal storm. Some parents then believe they are experiencing the "baby blues", but make no mistake: the baby blues is a postpartum depression, while the fatigue, stress and annoyances experienced in just 3 to 5 days at the maternity are not bearable, most of all for a woman subjected to the hormonal storm. Conscious of these conditions, which seem to affect a very large proportion of young mothers, some parents opt for smaller institutions where the follow-up will be more benevolent and less impersonal, or for more natural methods. Whatever the birth plan or the means of the parents, it is important to keep in mind that the essential remains the well-being of the parents and the baby, the mother's rest, and the serenity given to the baby. Parents can limit the visits of their relatives, make the choice to be the least disturbed possible, change their environment to make it more serene (for example: ask for an extra bed for the father, bring the favorite snacks of the mother, use relatives' visiting to ask them to bring something, etc.), apply certain techniques to rest while reassuring the child, such as massage, portering, skin-to-skin (which, moreover, will allow the child to learn to regulate his body temperature more quickly, will put him to sleep more quickly, decrease his crying, allow him a fast mental and motor development, and increase the lactation of the mother), or the co-sleeping. In general, baby's development issues arise from pregnancy and will allow you to choose what techniques to adopt in the womb.

Notes

Optional course 2: The pregnant woman's diet

Foods to advise

The nutrient requirements of pregnant women change significantly during pregnancy. Especially in terms of vitamins, the growth of the baby leads to consumption peaks that will cause the mother herself to consume rich foods:

- 1st trimester: vitamin B and iron
- 2nd trimester: calcium
- In the 3rd trimester: in vitamin A

In general, the diet of the pregnant woman must be healthy, rich and varied. And include mainly raw and cooked fiber, protein, fruit and vegetables (well cleaned in several vinegar baths), oily fish, lean meats and dairy products (equivalent to at least ½ liter of milk a day).

Pace

The pregnant woman is often embarrassed at the intestinal level, and sometimes even weakened according to the trimester or the pathological state of the pregnancy. It is important to find your rhythm, even if you have many small, slow meals during the day. Eating little but often can indeed allow you to ensure a continuous energy level and an optimal diet for your baby. If needed, dietary supplements may be prescribed by your doctor, obstetrician or midwife.

Foods to avoid

The risks of toxoplasmosis and listeriosis make it necessary to limit the consumption of red meat and to eat it well cooked. Similarly, the raw vegetables must be well cleaned (in several vinegar water baths) and the raw fish must be avoided or consumed by having previously frozen in order to neutralize the possible pathogenic organisms. Foods based on raw milk (cheese ...) must be removed in favor of those based on pasteurized milk.

For breastfeeding

To prepare for breastfeeding, you can promote dairy products, starchy foods and all types of fruits and vegetables, starting with fennel that is lactogenic and raw carrots. Oily fish are excellent sources of vitamins and proteins. Finally, during breastfeeding, cabbages and similar (cauliflower, broccoli ...) should be avoided to limit the risk of colic in infants. Mint is forbidden unless you want to stop breastfeeding because it is a powerful inhibitor.

Alcohol, tobacco, drugs

Alcohol, tobacco and all other psychotropic substances are of course to be banned during pregnancy and breastfeeding. The risks to your infant are not yet all identified, so if your addiction is too strong, we recommend that you be followed and helped to stop.

Notes

Optional course 3 : Suitcase for maternity

Maternity clinics often offer a list or a trousseau to take with you so that the stay is comfortable. Most of the time, these lists are very exhaustive, and most of the young mothers state that they have not used half of the objects carried away and that they would reconsider most of the quantities afterwards. On the other hand, certain elements are forgotten, for example the father's suitcase, which, even if he does not necessarily stay at the maternity ward with his wife, will nevertheless spend many hours there. Here are standard lists, revised according to actual needs for the delivery room and a 4-day stay at the maternity ward. We specify that it is necessary to differentiate for each, a bag that will follow you in the delivery room, a suitcase that will contain all your effects for a stay in a maternity room.

Delivery room: Mother's bag

✓ a copy of your birthing plan
✓ a lightweight dressing gown and cosy slippers
✓ a nightshirt or a big T-shirt to wear while in labour
✓ bathrobe and towel
✓ socks, feet can get cold during labour
✓ massage oil, if you'd like to be massaged during labour
✓ lip balm and water atomizer

✓ The big T-shirt or nightgown will be worn during labor and possibly delivery: so plan for a garment in which you feel comfortable and that will allow the legs to be widened as needed. Avoid shorts or pants that tighten in the abdomen and that will become difficult to withstand during contractions.
✓ The bathrobe and towel will be useful when giving birth in the pool, or shower during work to better withstand contractions
✓ The atomizer may be indicated as optional, but is usually brought by all future mothers, because it allows you to get hydrated during labor and delivery, which can be of great help to you, since you do not have have the right to eat or drink while working and giving birth.

Delivery room: Baby's bag

- ✓ pajama or sleepsuit and vest
- ✓ a body
- ✓ baby blanket
- ✓ a hat
- ✓ pair of socks
- ✓ sleeping bag
- ✓ bath towel

✓ The body and the pajamas go together. If you opt for this set of clothes, the bra and socks will be useless. And conversely if you opt for the bra and socks that will allow you to warm the baby on areas that will not come into contact skin-to-skin if you decide to do. In general, all clothing is to be taken in size 1 month (54 cm), the birth size (50 cm) can be small if the baby comes to term. The last ultrasound at 32 weeks (8 months) will give you an idea of how big your baby will be when he or she leaves. The cap is always necessary because the newborn does not yet know how to regulate the temperature of his head. Finally, if you decide to take a skin-to-skin T-shirt or headband, be aware that most of the items listed above will be useless, but that you should still have them available in the event of unforeseen circumstances during your delivery (for example, emergency cesarean section).

✓ The bath towel will be used for infant first aid while the young mother will receive postpartum care herself.

✓ The fitted sheet and blanket will be used to prepare the baby's cradle. The blanket is not necessary but it can be used, put under the cover sheet, to reproduce a cocoon for the comfort of your baby.

✓ The sleeping bag must be chosen according to the season and the size of the baby (here sizes of 0 to 3 months are suitable). Parents are advised to choose a sleeveless sleeping bag, with snap-on straps, and a zip to open it completely, which will simplify its use.

Delivery room: Dad's bag

If the Dad comes to accompany the future mother in his work until his delivery, he can guess that he will potentially spend hours at the maternity ward. According to his involvement in the work of the mother, he will have a lot to do, or a lot of waiting. He will have to provide food, hydrate and wait. He can also, if the wait is long during the work, take something to change the ideas as well as those of the future mother, such as reading, music or videos. It could also entertain the future mother during her work and make the wait more bearable. Some future dads who accompany their wife or partner wish to avoid eating or drinking in solidarity with the mother. However, they must know that if they accompany the mother-to-be during their delivery, they may be very much in demand, especially in the delivery positions that require them to maintain a prolonged effort (for example, a dad may have to support his wife during her effort, while pulling her legs, an effort to maintain thrust and traction, throughout the duration of delivery, between 15 minutes and 1 hour). This requires a lot of physical presence, so it is recommended that they take strength, even discreetly out of solidarity for the young mother.

> ✓ snacks and drinks
> ✓ cash
> ✓ books and magazines
> ✓ a change of clothes
> ✓ mobile phone and charger
> ✓ a camera

✓ Replacement clothing will be useful in case of water loss if it helps the expectant mother during work or prolonged effort requiring change of clothes.
✓ The bathrobe and towel will be useful if the future dad accompanies the future mother in the pool.

Maternity stay: mom's suitcase

The stay in maternity lasts between 3 and 5 full days. The expectant mother will have to provide clothes and toiletries according to this duration. In addition, the mother will undergo care and will often be bedridden. It will therefore be necessary for it to choose loose and comfortable clothes, type pajamas or indoor relaxing outfits. For the breastfeeding mother, it is a question of providing breastfeeding or unbuttoned tops (shirts) and some breastfeeding discs when the rise of milk is in place (if the young mother opts for disposable breastfeeding pads, in provide one pair per day). Also provide bath towels, which are not always provided. Finally, you must know that your uterus is regenerating, you will have high blood loss in the first days and will decrease in the month following delivery. It is therefore necessary to provide a covering lingerie, natural material and easy to boil in case of traces of blood, cotton type, as well as thick sanitary napkins and very absorbent. Some clinics advise taking disposable underpants. In this case, take a size above yours because the sanitary napkins you will need will be very cumbersome. When it comes to personal hygiene, make sure that your personal gel is very respectful of the mucous membranes.

- ✓ travel toiletries
- ✓ two pairs of pyjamas with front-opening tops for easy feeding
- ✓ bath towels
- ✓ nursing pillow
- ✓ breast pads
- ✓ lanolin nipple cream
- ✓ maternity sanitary towels
- ✓ a pair of socks or slippers
- ✓ comfy going-home clothes

✓ The breastfeeding pillow is not needed if you want to lighten up and learn to breastfeed without using this type of cushion. It requires a particular learning, especially depending on the models and can therefore be very useful. Depending on the use you want to make, it may eventually be replaced by a bolster.

✓ To help breastfeeding, in case of slow or difficult milk rise, you can plan in advance to take food supplements favoring the production of milk powder to put in solution, capsules of fenugreek or yeast or homeopathy. You can also ask your doctor in advance to prescribe the rental of a breast pump that you can use while your baby is sleeping or just before feeding to activate your lactation. Hydration will greatly increase your milk production, so if the clinic does not provide you with it, arm yourself with bottled water. Adapted massage can also promote lactation while resolving any kind of pain.

Maternity stay: baby's suitcase

The maternity bag of the baby is overall the most complex to make, and also the most consistent, especially for a first child, when young parents have no benchmarks yet. In general, everything related to exchange will be taken in duplicate to avoid discomfort for parents who make their first exchange experiences and ensure maximum hygiene to the newborn. If you want to lighten up and you can rely on someone (potentially the father) to bring spare parts, especially cotton diapers or squares, you can build a home stock (which will be needed anyway from your return) and renew your stock at the mid-term maternity hospital. Plan an average of 2 packages of 80 cotton squares and 2 packs of 25 layers for the total length of stay.

For infant clothing, if you opt for skin-to-skin, your headband or t-shirt will be enough for you. Take a pair of bodysuits and pajamas in size 1 month in case of any need. For bodysuits, prefer kimono style bodysuits, easier to handle and more covering, pure cotton. For pajamas, fully-working models may be preferable if you're new to the game, then you'll probably prefer back-opening models when you're comfortable with the change. The bras will only be useful if you are skin-to-skin, then prefer the pure wool or pure wool jackets or jackets that will allow your baby to regulate while not attacking his fragile skin.

- ✓ two or three sleepsuits and vests
- ✓ newborn nappies and nappy bags
- ✓ newborn-friendly baby wipes
- ✓ a baby blanket
- ✓ sleeping bag
- ✓ swaddles and bibs
- ✓ some going-home clothes. An all-in-one outfit, cardigan, hat, socks and booties
- ✓ baby toiletries including a brush

- ✓ The swaddles and bibs are only useful when using the bottle and will be very little soiled.
- ✓ For the blanket and sleeping bag, the quantities are doubled in case of heavy soiling, which happens very little. If you have already provided a fitted sheet and a sleeping bag for the delivery room bag, take only one additional set. Prefer the use of the sleeping bag rather than bedding which increases the chances of choking when the baby is growing up.
- ✓ For the first days of the baby, the diapers will be useless, and the fitted sheet will not need to be protected, unless the layers are not properly installed. Subsequently, and as soon as you come home, the swaddling clothes will prove very useful.

74

✓ When choosing a brush for your baby, choose it with natural and soft bristles.

✓ For the choice of diapers, few washable diapers are adapted to the size of the infant. The washable diapers said to be adaptable in size from 0 years will not be suitable, unless your baby is already of a substantial size. If you opt, at least for the stay in maternity, for disposable diapers, know that most major brands use toxic products reinforcing the risk of infection of the skin of your baby: it is recommended that you inquire with consumer associations and check the compositions of the layers.

Maternity stay: dad's suitcase

Dad will be able to take, if he wishes to share the stay in maternity of his wife, the business that he usually takes for 4 to 5 days of vacation. He can also provide snacks for him and the young mother. In addition, during the stay at the maternity ward, he will have several opportunities to go out to declare the child to the registry office, purchase the prescribed care or make a payment of fees that will also allow him to make some food or others for the couple.

Notes

Optional course 4: choice of equipment

Among the wide variety of equipment choices that young parents can encounter, it is easy enough to get lost, and equipment that is supposed to simplify their parenting role can quickly become uncomfortable and cumbersome. It is therefore important to start with what you think is essential in your daily life, but especially how you want to live your parenting with your baby (proximity, mode of awakening and education, environment, childcare, etc. .) then step by step go to detail, going through the constraints and comfort, which will allow you to make a selection by elimination as in the figure below in the example:

Emily and James are scared by the size of this equipment. It must be said that they live in a 50 m² in the city center and have little space, that public transport is so efficient that they have never had a car ... and that they learn from pregnancy on the benefits of carrying and wrapping a baby that they would like to try. Moreover, if they had to define themselves in terms of parenthood, they would rather see themselves as " materning parents ", and give much importance to their proximity to their child. It is therefore clear that concerning them, a trio stroller will be of no use. In their case, it would be better to invest in an effective and ergonomic carrying solution, and why not some courses of portage and physiological exchanges with the baby. The question of the stroller will arise when the baby is old enough to go in a stroller, that is to say around 6 months, and if the parents start to find it heavy and wish to walk without getting too tired. They can then use a stroller cane, comfortable, inexpensive and space-saving.

Values: the way you have decided to live your parenting

Constraints: home, space, daily habits, transportation, etc.

Desiderata: functionnality choice with and for baby

Comfort: equipment you prefer (organisation, colours, etc.)

Another example:

Emma and Peter live in the countryside. Their numerous trips by car and their long walks in the forest made them immediately choose an off-road trio stroller. They have a lot of room and have already planned to make a room for their baby, but think that breastfeeding would be easier, especially at night, if their little angel spent his first months in their room. A baby room is easily furnished, but how to ensure the cohabitation with the baby in the room of the parents? Young parents want temporary, but only if it is comfortable for them and their baby. They therefore opt for a cradle in cododo easily convertible into a bed when the baby leaves the parental room. And decide not to clutter too much, to reconvert for a while the desk and its shelf at a changing table, on which they have the changing mat of the baby and organize diapers and care products.

Transportation

The question of transport is quite easy following the previous diagram: it depends a lot on whether you have a car or not. If this is the case, a cozy adapted from birth and meeting safety standards is recommended, or a nacelle for long trips. This kind of equipment is also very easy to fit on a stroller when buying a duo or trio stroller. Check comfort for your baby and adaptability by car. In addition, some brands are prohibitively expensive because of their notoriety, so do not hesitate to study the second hand market or follow the cycles of promotions and bargains in specialty shops. If you are a fan of portage because ideal for the psychomotor development of the baby, do not hesitate to invest in a comfortable and ergonomic baby carrier, especially if you want to wear your baby for a long time and if the perineum of the mother is not still re-educated. For the first few months, the T-shirt and skin-to-skin carrier bagging solution is an excellent substitute for the baby carrier, which requires special equipment.

House

In addition to the rooms where the baby will spend his days and will have a dedicated space (toys, deckchair - more comfortable than the cozy for long periods and can potentially follow you in each room if it is equipped with handles or substitute a cradle if it includes the inclined position, wake-up mat, mobile, etc., your house will have to be secured little by little when your baby starts to move on its own, between 6 months and 1 year for the walk to four legs, until standing up. For the bath of your baby you will need to provide a bath in your bathroom (if you have little space, the inflatable bath is very comfortable and foldable bathtubs are also a very compact solution). Finally, if you give the bottle, your kitchen should have a dedicated corner including drainer, brushes, storage space and what to prepare the bottles. It can also serve as kitchen space to prepare your baby's jar from 6 months, when you decide to diversify his food.

Bedroom

You may decide to prepare a room for the baby in advance. This kind of project can accompany the future parents in the preparation for their future role and take the path of parenthood. However, it is not advisable to leave your baby alone in your room before your third month: indeed, the baby is considered as infant during the first 3 months and needs to be reassured by the presence of his parents. In addition, most babies sleep 6 hours from 3 or 4 months and keeping them close to you, especially in cododo, can not have to get up several times in the night. Some parents even opt for technical solutions that allow the infant to sleep directly in their own bed, but this is not recommended by midwives, especially if you want to take time as a couple. The baby's room usually has a crib or crib, a changing table, a wardrobe to store clothes and a play area. It is recommended to decorate the room with soft colors and in places, contrasting patterns, mobile, etc. In addition, this room must be secure so that the child avoids hurting himself when he moves alone.

Notes

Optional course 5: Infant care

Although the way in which taking care of their baby seems to worry most new moms, preparation from pregnancy and motherhood learning, good exercise and good practice lay the foundation for parenting expertise, as well as training. By the repetition of gestures, it will also consolidate.

Change

Change experience is most frequently repeated for parents, since a newborn is changed between 8 and 12 times in 24 hours, and then as the child develops and the regularity of his life changes the digestive tract, the number of changes will gradually decrease between 5 and 8 per day. The change may seem impressive to parents the first time: learning to place the baby on the changing table, hold it while cleaning, use the products, put back the diaper, are gestures that parents will learn both to quickly master. In order to make learning more effective and enjoyable, it is recommended that parents change the baby together for the first time: this will allow them to visualize the organization they will have to set up to change the baby serenely when each of them is alone, while helping each other for the first time. We recommend organizing the space and defining the roles before each exchange experience. For the first days at the maternity ward, the meconium, very sticky to the skin of the infant, will be more easily removed with hot water, then it will dry the baby's skin by dabbing gently with a cotton square before apply oleo-limestone liniment with another square of cotton. In general, water and liniment oleo-limestone are the best friends of the exchange. Be careful to prefer organic products and non-toxic especially if the skin of your baby is sensitive or atopic tendency. For this purpose, the wipes are not recommended and can, even during travel, be replaced by cotton squares and a small bottle of water. In the same way, only certain brands of layers are identified as non-toxic. We therefore advise young parents to get information from consumer associations.

Bath

The bath can be given to infants every 2 days because they do not get so dirty in the beginning and their skin is very sensitive. It is even advisable for parents of babies whose skin is atopic or if an eczema is declared in one of the parents, to wash their baby once every 3 days or once a week if an eczema is declared at the child, choosing products with a neutral pH. The temperature of the bath should be controlled with a bath thermometer and should be around 37 ° C. The first baths with the baby must be short to prevent him from losing his body temperature, from 1 to 2 minutes and will lengthen with the passing of the months when the bigger baby, will have pleasure to take his bath, without exceeding the 10 minutes . Drying should be short and effective by wrapping your baby in a towel or bath towel and tapping gently to mop the water. Never rub your fragile skin, or forget to dry inside the folds, which will appear especially when your baby will grow, which can be a source of infection.

Cord care

During its first 10 days of life, the baby will have an ersatz umbilical cord that will dry before falling leaving room for the belly button. To prevent infection and help the cord dry out, it should be disinfected from the base upwards and the dried blood removed with mild disinfectant suitable for infants and a sterile compress. This operation can be repeated 2 to 3 a day.

Nose wiping and cleaning the eyes

If necessary, your baby can be bled (usually, this is not necessary because the baby clears the mucus while sneezing) being positioned ¾ on the stomach. This is to put a small splash of saline into the highest nostril (closest to you), then close it with your finger. The baby will naturally eject the serum by blowing through the other nostril. Turn the baby and then repeat the gesture on the other nostril.

Your baby may also need you to clean his eyes. This is to put a few drops of saline on the four corners of a sterile compress: use the first corner that you drag from the outside of the eye (closest to the ear) to the inside. Change the corner (you should never use the same corner to avoid the risk of infection), and drag it from the inside of the eye (closest to the nose) to the cheek. Change the corner and repeat the operation for the other eye.

Food supplements
Your baby will need vitamin D for at least his first year and vitamin K. These dietary supplements are often transmitted as drops and are given in the morning around feedings. Feel free to administer these supplements to two, if keeping the infant's head is too complicated to one hand.

Awakening
To allow the baby a good sensory and emotional development, it is advisable to massage regularly, especially after bathing or changing with sweet almond oil or coconut, or simply organic olive oil or liniment. This helps the development of touch, as well as caresses, especially during feedings, or kissing, especially when you wear your baby. For hearing, it is often talking to him in a

gentle and caring manner, which will allow him to reassure while learning to recognize the voices of those around him and develop the brain areas related to speech. Establishing a routine where you sing his song (the one you have chosen and that you will enjoy singing to him every day) also allows him a good development while reassuring him. The taste is developed by the mother's milk which takes the taste of what the mother eats, if the child is breastfed. About 1 to 2 months, you can start to make him feel food to develop his sense of smell. As for the sight, it is that of your smile that will reassure your child and teach him to gradually identify facial expressions. It should be remembered that the infant better identifies the contrasts, so presenting him with an expressive face will reassure him.

Notes

Because it is often difficult for future parents to prepare for a new birth, or to regain their reflexes when a newborn arrives within the family, this simple and concise guide inspired by the birth courses proposed in France, serves as an effective support for a serene preparation. It includes notes and tips from the experience of parents and professionals, as well as many images, examples and free pages to take your notes. This book is intended as a real support for childbirth preparation classes and can also be used by caregivers.

www.ingramcontent.com/pod-product-compliance
Lightning Source LLC
Chambersburg PA
CBHW041204180526
45172CB00006B/1184